From Binge to Balance

Undoing years of Hustle with one Healthy Habit at a time

Anupama Nair

BlueRose ONE
Stories Matter
NewDelhi • London

BLUEROSE PUBLISHERS
India | U.K.

For permissions requests or inquiries regarding this publication, please contact:

BLUEROSE PUBLISHERS
www.BlueRoseONE.com
info@bluerosepublishers.com
+91 8882 898 898
+4407342408967

ISBN: 978-93-7310-357-0

Cover Design: Aman Sharma
Typesetting: Manisha Rawat

First Edition: November 2025

Dedication

To God Almighty

for guiding me to my purpose, for revealing the mission I was meant to live, and for lighting the path even when I didn't know I was searching. Your grace has been my anchor.

To my tribe

My mother, the epitome of silent strength, whose resilience is etched in my soul.

My father, the disciplinarian especially when it comes to food.

My brother, who serves the nation with pride – a reflection of the values we were raised with.

My Father & Mother in-laws who always supported me.

My husband, who went to the gym on Day 1 of marriage and has never stopped pushing me to be stronger – physically, mentally, spiritually.

To my Mentor

And my daughter Anvi, my greatest teacher, my fiercest cheerleader, and my daily reminder of why I must show up – wiser, braver, and kinder.

This one's for you.

Foreword

When I first met Anupama, she wasn't just another nutritionist. She was a force – part coach, part cheerleader, part scientist, and part therapist (sometimes all within a single session).

She didn't just help me lose weight – she helped me gain something far more important: clarity, energy, and a sense of control over my health.

What makes this book powerful is that it's not written from theory. It's written from lived experience – hers, mine, and hundreds of others who've worked with her.

So, if you're holding this book, you're already halfway there. The rest? Flip the page, follow the breadcrumbs, and start your transformation.

– A real client, a real believer, and now a real friend.

Acknowledgments

This book would not have been possible without the real heroes of my transformation:

To my **clients** – thank you for trusting me not just with your health, but with your stories, struggles, and spreadsheets of food logs.

To my **inner circle of friends** – the ones who cheered even when I swapped laddoos for chia pudding.

To every person who ever thought *"I've tried everything"* – I see you, I was you. And I wrote this for you.

Thank you for walking this journey with me. This book is ours.

Preface

If someone had told me in my early 30s — back when I was skipping meals, skipping sleep, and skipping out on my own well-being — that I'd one day write a book on health, I would've laughed… and then probably ordered dessert. Twice.

But here I am.

This book is not just about food, fitness, or fat loss. It's about coming home — to your body, to your breath, and to your own inner wisdom. It's the blueprint I wish I had a decade ago, before the midnight Maggi, before the burnout, before the belly fat became a permanent accessory.

Whether you're a corporate leader, a tired mom, or someone stuck between weight-loss attempts #17 and #18 — this book is your permission slip to reset without regret.

Contents

PART I:
THE WAKE-UP CALL

Chapter 1

The Price of Success

My Early 30s: Late Nights, Quick Fix Meals, and the Hidden Cost of Hustle

My Early 30s: Late Nights, Quick Fix Meals, and the Hidden Cost of Hustle

I come from an army family — the kind where waking up before sunrise wasn't an act of heroism, it was just... normal. Polished shoes, perfectly pressed uniforms, a schedule so tight it could rival a Swiss train — that was everyday life. My father and mother, both now retired, lived by the clock. My brother, proudly serving now, has carried that baton forward — literally and figuratively. I still remember my dad sitting with his morning chai and newspaper at exactly 6:00 AM — not 5:59, not 6:01. Discipline wasn't a habit. It was oxygen.

And then, there's my mom — a force of nature. She retired as a Major General in the Military Nursing Services, and if there was ever a living definition of "self-made and unstoppable," it's her. Independent, fiercely determined, and unshakably committed to her work and family, she's been my role model from day one. From her, I learned that being a woman and being strong are not two separate things — they're the same thing.

My brother? Another powerhouse. His only and only aim in life was to join the Army. No plan B. No distractions. No "maybe later." He was so laser-focused that he shaped his entire life around that dream — and achieved it. Watching him chase his goal was like having a daily masterclass in persistence.

So yes — discipline, ambition, and determination were practically the family heirlooms I inherited.

And then I got married into a civilian household.

Now here's the twist — they didn't make me laid back. I did that all by myself. Somewhere along the way, I stopped prioritizing myself. My husband — bless him — went to the gym from day one of our marriage. Every. Single. Day. And me? I watched him with zero FOMO and a full bowl of popcorn. It didn't even occur to me to consider fitness. My mind was too full of to-do lists, client calls, and finding the right series to binge on.

Bit by bit, my precision army upbringing gave way to a life that looked more like a late-night startup founder's calendar — minus the unicorn funding or IPO dreams.

The Great Trade-off: Time vs. Health

My 30s were supposed to be the peak years — and they were — in every area except my health.

Up until my daughter was born, I was part of the corporate world. And let me be honest — it was never my calling. I never truly felt I belonged in that world; it was just something I did because... well, that's what you do, right? But when my daughter came into our lives, she gave me a new purpose. I took a conscious decision to step away from my regular job and be fully present for her.

It wasn't an easy decision — corporate paychecks are addictive — but I knew it was the right one. And unlike the stories I've heard so many times — *"After my firstborn, I put on 10 kilos, and my second one added another 10!"* or *"Since my delivery, my stomach has been hanging out"* — I can't blame motherhood for my body. I worked right until my delivery, didn't believe in "eating for two," gained only 11 kilos during pregnancy, and lost all of it within six months. So nope — my daughter didn't make me gain weight. My own lifestyle choices later did that job just fine.

With a full-time job replaced by full-time family responsibilities, and the constant pressure to be "on," I began to trade off nutritious meals for quick bites between Zoom calls and errands. Breakfast? Optional. Lunch? Usually cold. Dinner? At 11 PM, and often eaten while watching yet another show I'd never remember the name of.

What started as an "it's just a phase" became a full-blown lifestyle. And then it began to show — not just on the weighing scale, but on my skin, energy levels, and worst of all, my confidence.

Sleep: The First Casualty

Sleep hygiene? Forget hygiene – sleep itself was missing. Late-night scrolling, stress from work, and binge-watching "just one more episode" ensured that my body was sleep-deprived, cortisol-high, and silently inflamed. But I pushed through. That's what hustlers do, right?

Except – the body keeps the score. And mine started showing all the warning signs.

The weight wouldn't go. The cravings wouldn't stop. And I was TIRED. Always.

I remember staring at myself in the mirror one morning – face bloated, under eyes puffy, and stomach feeling like it had a second personality. That's when I knew something had to change. But I didn't know what yet.

What I did know was this – I couldn't spend the next 30 years like this and expect to retire into my best life. Something had to give. And this time, it wouldn't be my health.

"You can't pour from an empty cup – especially if it's full of caffeine and sugar."

That realization set me on a journey I never imagined – a journey that took me from carb-loading to keto-cooking, from skipping meals to structured fasting, and from fearing weights to running marathons. And no, I still don't look like Arnold.

(But my arms? They do deserve some flexing.)

Chapter 2

When the Body Says No

Fatigue, Inflammation, Brain Fog – How I Ignored the Signs Until I Couldn't

You know those warning lights that flash on your car dashboard? The ones you pretend not to see because you're already late and convincing yourself that it's just the air freshener sensor acting up?

That was me – **but with my own body.**

My body was flashing **every red signal possible** – fatigue, random aches, bloating that made me look six months pregnant by 6 PM, mood swings that even I couldn't keep up with, and brain fog so bad I once forgot my laptop password, ATM pin, and my own birthday… all in one day.

Energy? Never Heard of Her

Let's talk about fatigue. Not the "I had a long day" kind of tired – I'm talking about "why-does-my-soul-feel-heavy" kind of exhaustion.

I would wake up feeling tired, like I had wrestled a baby elephant in my dreams. Post-lunch was a predictable crash, and evening energy? Only available if you count lying down dramatically and asking existential questions like, "Why am I like this?"

And the worst part? I found it hard to be fully present in my daughter's life. I was so tired that picking her up often felt like a workout I wasn't ready for. My lower back would ache, my arms would cramp, and I'd feel trapped in my own body – not able to do the very things I wanted to do as a mother. That hurt more than the physical pain itself.

And yes, I still had a full-time job, family duties, and the occasional social event where I'd dress up, click pictures, and crash by 9 PM like I had just run a marathon. (Back then, I didn't know I'd actually run marathons someday. Life's funny.)

The Mystery of the Disappearing Waistline

Despite doing "everything right" (in my opinion), the weight refused to budge. And not just that – my waistline was slowly but steadily making plans to meet my chest.

I blamed water retention, the moon cycle, slow metabolism, gluten, the weather, and my neighbor's negative vibes. Everything – except my lifestyle.

Meanwhile, clothes that once fit like a dream were now acting like I had betrayed them. I once tried wearing an old kurta and it let out a sound I can only describe as fabric panic.

Skin, Gut & Other Betrayals

Let's not even get started on my skin. Patches. Breakouts. Puffiness. Under-eye circles that could qualify for solar eclipses.

The gut? Always in chaos. One day constipated, the next day a digestive rollercoaster. I was either popping saunf, ginger tea, or googling "how to reset your stomach overnight."

Every specialist I visited gave me a list of tests and told me: **"You just need rest and a better routine."** Thanks, Doc. Do you also do magic?

And Then Came Brain Fog

Imagine this: I'd open the fridge, stare for five minutes, and still forget why I came. I'd walk into rooms with purpose, and exit with... nothing.

Multitasking was no longer a flex — it was a trap. My mind felt like 100 open tabs in Chrome with Spotify playing random songs in the background. And somewhere, an update reminder just kept blinking: "Please restart your system."

But I Ignored It All

Because "I'm just busy."

Because "This is normal after 30."

Because "Everyone feels this way."

Because... **I didn't know any better.**

Until one day — during a client meeting — I forgot what I was saying halfway through the sentence. I laughed it off, blaming 'mommy brain' and 'sleep debt.' But inside? I panicked.

Because when your body whispers and you don't listen – it starts screaming.

And mine was yelling: "WAKE UP, WOMAN!"

It wasn't just weight. It was inflammation, insulin resistance, a broken circadian rhythm, and a seriously messed-up gut microbiome. Of course, I didn't know all those fancy terms back then. All I knew was – I couldn't keep living like this.

Something had to change.

Not temporarily. Not for a vacation or a photoshoot. But for life.

That was the turning point. The moment I decided to go from being a silent sufferer to a conscious warrior. Not with another fad, but with **deep, slow, sustainable shifts.**

I didn't know where to begin – but I knew I wasn't going back.

"Your body doesn't betray you. It warns you."

I had finally started listening.

Chapter 3
Searching for the Way Out

Why Diets Failed Me and What Finally Made Me Take Responsibility

At some point in your 30s, after enough bloating, brain fog, and bathroom drama, you realize that maybe — just maybe — the answer isn't another "3-day detox challenge" you found on Instagram.

But before that realization hits, you go on a wild ride.

And oh boy, did I ride all the rides.

My Tour of Failed Diets

Let's start with the **Soup Cleanse**.

Whoever said soup is comforting clearly never drank cold cabbage broth for three days while everyone else at home ordered pizza. I lost two kilos and my will to live.

Then there was the **Raw Food Phase**.

It sounded earthy and spiritual — until I chewed carrots so much my jaw started sounding like bubble wrap.

The GM Diet?

Let's just say Day 4 (bananas and milk) nearly broke me. I haven't looked at bananas the same way since.

I also tried low-fat everything.

Because clearly, fat was the villain, right? So I filled my kitchen with fat-free biscuits, fat-free yogurt, and fat-free snacks — which were basically sugar bombs wearing a halo.

And let's not forget **juice fasting**.

My body didn't know what hit it. Day 2 felt like my organs were calling HR to report me.

Yet, every time the scale showed even a hint of movement, I would declare the diet a success. Until, of course, I blinked... and all the weight came back with interest. Like it had been on a quick vacation and returned with friends.

The Excuse Olympics

During this phase, I also became a gold medalist in excuses.

"I don't have time to meal prep."

"I deserve a reward after this stressful week."

"I'll start Monday."

"Wait — is mercury in retrograde?"

I blamed everything – my genes, my job, my schedule, the weather, and even the emotional trauma of watching that one K-drama.

Responsibility? Never even met her.

Then Came The Mirror Moment

One day, I stood in front of the mirror wearing my "slightly tight" jeans (they had now become "don't breathe too hard" jeans), and thought:

"How many more shortcuts am I going to take before I actually figure this out?"

It wasn't about being slim anymore.

It was about **feeling like myself again**. Energetic. Focused. Light.

Not just for a wedding or a vacation – but every single day.

And there it was – the aha moment.

No fairy god-nutritionist. No magic pill. Just a quiet, uncomfortable truth:

"Maybe I need to stop outsourcing my health to diet plans and start taking charge."

So, I did something revolutionary.

I stopped looking for the next "quick fix"...

...and started looking for **myself**.

Taking Responsibility (with a Side of Sarcasm)

Taking responsibility wasn't dramatic. I didn't burn all my chips or cry into a salad.

It was more like this internal eye-roll where I said,

"Okay, fine. I created this chaos — now let's fix it."

I started learning. I stopped blindly following trends.

I listened to my mentors. I read real science.

And I asked myself — not "what will make me lose 5 kgs by Friday" — but **"what will support me for life?"**

Spoiler alert: The answer wasn't cabbage soup.

"You can't heal your body with punishment. But you can heal it with ownership."

And that's where things began to change.

Not overnight, not dramatically — but deeply.

Step by step, I started building a foundation.

No more food guilt. No more rollercoasters.

Just a steady shift from "what's the next diet?" to "what does my body need today?"

And finally... I started heading in the right direction.

PART II:
THE EXPERIMENTATION PHASE

Chapter 4

Keto – The Good, The Bad, and The Butter

How I Burned Fat, Rewired My Brain, and Made Friends with Ghee

If you've ever typed "how to lose weight quickly" into Google, you've probably come across a magical four-letter word: **KETO**.

At first glance, it sounds like a stylish new Japanese restaurant.

"Where are we dining tonight?"

"Oh, just this new place in town called Keto! Very high-end, lots of fats, no rice."

But little did I know, Keto wasn't a restaurant — it was an entire **lifestyle**.

And the first time I actually understood what keto really meant — not just in a Pinterest-recipe sense — was when I met **Kaizzad Capadia Sir**, the man who would become my mentor, myth-buster, and fitness reality check all rolled into one.

Meeting the Man Who Walked the Talk

It was at K11 School of Fitness Sciences – a place I had nervously walked into, half expecting protein shakes to fall from the ceiling.

Then I met him.

Kaizzad Capadia Sir – the Director, Founder, Principal, and most importantly, the human version of Google Search (minus the pop-ups).

He didn't just talk about fitness. **He lived it.**

Every word, every principle, every rep – he embodied the discipline and strength most people only post about on Instagram.

What struck me first wasn't just his physique (though, hello!) – it was his **clarity**.

No fluff, no fancy jargon – just deep, powerful truths delivered with brutal honesty and surgical precision.

And you know what?

He **never sold shortcuts.**

He taught principles – metabolism, insulin response, bio-individuality – things that made me realize I'd spent most of my adult life listening to influencers who barely knew how digestion worked.

Kaizzad Sir wasn't here to flatter egos. He was here to educate. And that... inspired me deeply.

In a world full of noise, he was a lighthouse.

Keto: Not Just Butter Coffee and Bacon

Through his teachings and my own rabbit-hole research, I discovered that **KETO was not a "diet."**

It wasn't about eating cheese cubes like popcorn or wrapping everything in bacon.

It was a science-backed, metabolic strategy.

I learned that when you reduce carbs significantly, your body flips a metabolic switch.

Instead of using glucose (sugar) as its primary fuel, it starts burning **fat** for energy – through a process called ketosis.

Yes, you read that right.

My body – which had spent years hoarding fat like a squirrel in winter – was now **using it as fuel.**

It was like convincing your bank to pay you for all the debt you collected. Wild, right?

The Good: Fat for the Win

Once I crossed the "carb withdrawal" phase (more on that in a bit), something amazing happened.

I felt… **awake**.

Mentally sharp. Like I had cleaned the foggy windshield of my brain.

No more post-lunch crashes.

No more "hanger" fits over evening snacks.

And best of all – **steady fat loss.**

I could see my body transforming in ways no juice cleanse had ever managed.

My skin cleared up. Energy soared. People started asking what "treatment" I was on.

(Answer: Paneer sautéed in ghee. Doctor approved.)

The Bad: Keto Flu and Cauliflower Pizza Lies

Let's not pretend keto was all smooth sailing.

Week one felt like I was being ghosted by sugar and carbs at the same time.

Headaches. Mood swings. Cravings so intense, I would've happily traded my house for one warm spoon of jeera rice.

Then came the keto-friendly imposters – the foods that promised joy but delivered betrayal.

Cauliflower crust pizza? False hope in a circular shape.

Keto ice cream? More like frozen disappointment.

Almond flour bread? Let's just say it made a better coaster than a sandwich.

But despite the culinary heartbreak, I soldiered on.

Because when Kaizzad Sir said something was right for the body — I followed without a second thought.

If he said ghee is good, I stopped questioning and started pouring.

If he said "this is what your metabolism needs", I trusted him. No Googling. No second-guessing. Just surrender and action.

His voice became my compass in the chaos of conflicting nutrition advice.

"You don't change your body with motivation. You change it with commitment."

Those words were my fuel on the tough days.

So I committed.

Cooked my own meals. Cut the noise.

And slowly — keto stopped being a "diet" I was trying, and became a foundation I was living.

The Misunderstood Macros

Let's clear something up — Keto isn't a cheese buffet or a bacon party.

And it certainly isn't about turning every meal into a butter sculpture.

But I didn't have to overthink it — because I had someone who already walked the walk.

I simply followed what Kaizzad Sir taught: Eat real, whole foods. Respect fat. Keep carbs minimal. Listen to your body.

No macro calculators. No influencer hacks. Just fundamentals, taught with conviction and clarity.

It wasn't about "high fat" like samosas and pakoras on repeat.

It was about high-quality fats – like ghee, avocado, nuts, and coconut oil – combined with moderate protein and low carbs.

And once I started following this rhythm, the results followed me.

Most importantly, I began to reconnect with my body – tuning into hunger, fullness, energy, and mood – things I hadn't noticed in years.

Keto didn't just change how I ate – it changed how I listened to myself.

The Butter Revelation

If I had to summarize keto in one moment, it was the first time I added **butter to my coffee**.

I remember sipping it, raising an eyebrow, and thinking:

"This is either a nutrition breakthrough... or a sign of a midlife crisis."

Turns out, it was both.

That keto phase laid my **metabolic foundation**.

It taught me to respect food, question everything I thought I knew, and listen to my body.

And though I eventually transitioned into intermittent fasting as a more sustainable rhythm – keto was my gateway into **metabolic freedom.**

"Keto taught me that fat isn't the enemy. Confusion is."

Chapter 5
Beyond the Scale

Mental Clarity, Blood Work, and Non-Scale Victories I Didn't Expect

Let's admit it – when most of us start a diet or new lifestyle, our relationship with the weighing scale becomes borderline obsessive.

You wake up, pee (because every gram counts), remove all unnecessary clothing (bye-bye rubber band), step on the scale, hold your breath like that burns calories – and pray.

"Please... please show me some mercy."

And when it doesn't budge?

You spiral.

"I worked so hard! I said no to cake! I drank green sludge! What more do you want from me?!"

Been there. Cried there. Weighed myself again an hour later just in case the fat fairy had made a surprise visit.

But here's the twist:

When I finally stopped chasing the number and started focusing on **health**, something magical happened — victories started showing up in places I wasn't even looking.

Victory #1: Mental Clarity - Who Needs Google Calendar?

Suddenly, I could think clearly.

No more walking into rooms and forgetting why I was there.

No more rereading the same email six times.

No more mistaking my daughter's science project for a snack because I was running on 2 hours of sleep and 8 spoons of sugar.

It was like the fog in my brain lifted and my neurons finally showed up to work.

I went from "Where did I put my phone?" to "Let me tell you the Wi-Fi password, blood test ranges, and my grocery list from memory."

This was the moment I realized that food isn't just fuel for the body — it's software for the brain.

Victory #2: The Blood Report Didn't Come with a Lecture

You know you're getting healthy when your lab technician stops looking at you with sympathy.

My first "before" blood report looked like a sad song.

Vitamin D? Low.

Insulin? High.

Cholesterol? Confused.

But after a few months of real food, fasting, and not treating every evening like a buffet rehearsal, my blood reports began behaving.

My doctor even smiled – a first in 10 years.

He said, "This is good progress."

And I almost cried.

Because for once, the conversation wasn't about medicine – it was about momentum.

Victory #3: Clothes That Zipped Without Prayers

There's a special kind of happiness that comes when your favorite jeans **just fit** – no deep squats, no laying on the bed, no sucking in air like you're about to dive underwater.

I opened my cupboard and started rediscovering clothes I had mentally donated to the "maybe someday" pile.

And each time something slid on without resistance, I did a small victory dance (low impact, high joy).

The scale hadn't moved drastically – but my **body had changed.**

And that was all that mattered.

Victory #4: Energy That Didn't Need Coffee to Exist

Before, I lived on caffeine.

Morning coffee to wake up.

Mid-morning coffee to stay up.

Evening coffee so I could crash into bed at 1 AM and wonder why I couldn't sleep.

Now? I wake up with energy. Like, actual energy. From my own cells. Not beans.

It was so unfamiliar that I questioned it.

"Is this... health? Is this what people meant when they said 'I feel great'?"

I thought they were lying. But no — it's real.

I no longer felt like I needed a 3-day vacation after doing groceries. My body could finally keep up with my to-do list — and sometimes, even outrun it.

Victory #5: Confidence, the Quiet Kind

The biggest win wasn't even physical.

It was waking up and not dreading the mirror.

It was going for a walk not because I "had to burn calories," but because it felt good.

It was choosing meals based on what nourished me, not what punished me.

I wasn't chasing a size anymore.

I was reclaiming a state of being.

One where I felt strong, light, and... me.

"Health isn't just measured in kilos. It's measured in how brightly you live your life."

So, if you're stuck on the scale, waiting for it to give you permission to celebrate – let me be your permission slip.

Look at your skin. Your sleep. Your strength. Your stamina.

And the way you say "no" to nonsense with a smile now.

That's progress. And that's worth everything.

Chapter 6

From Frequent Feeder to Fat Burner

The Unexpected Superpower of Skipping Meals (and Surviving a Pandemic)

Now listen – I'm a creature of habit.

I love my comfort zone.

I love my high-fat, low-carb life.

I love the sound of ghee sizzling in a pan.

And yes, I loved eating at regular intervals – especially the kind that included post-workout smoothies, protein laddoos, and the occasional emotional snack that "just happened."

So you can imagine my reaction when, one fine 2018 morning – somewhere between sipping warm lemon water and planning my breakfast – my husband walked up to me, looked unusually serious, and said:

"Let's try intermittent fasting."

I blinked.

I laughed.

I checked if he was feverish.

Because what he *actually* said to me, in my head, translated to:

"Let's starve voluntarily and smile while doing it."

My Initial Reaction: Protein Panic

"Fasting?" I gasped, clutching my protein shaker like it was a life raft.

"How will I train without food? What about my post-workout protein? Won't my muscles just pack up and leave? What if I faint mid-squat and they have to call the gym trainer to drag me out?"

This man clearly didn't understand the sacred gym-fuel relationship.

But he had that calm confidence – the kind that's both charming and annoying when you're spiraling – and said:

"Just try it. Worst case, we'll stop."

Famous last words.

Intermittent What Now?

So I did what any rational human would do before skipping breakfast:

I Googled.

Turns out intermittent fasting isn't a new-age cult. It's actually a science-backed, time-restricted eating pattern that helps:

regulate insulin

improve fat burn

and give your digestive system a well-deserved break.

We started with the classic **16:8** –

16 hours of fasting, 8 hours of eating.

I still got my two meals. I still had coffee. I just didn't graze like a hamster all day.

And shockingly – I didn't faint. I didn't lose muscle.

Instead, I felt like a **metabolic ninja.**

The First Week: An Emotional Rollercoaster

Day 1: I sighed every 8 minutes, "Is it 1 PM yet?"

Day 2: I smelled food from two floors away and identified spice blends like a bloodhound.

Day 3: I Googled "How long before your body eats itself?"

Day 5: I felt light. Focused. In control.

Working Out Fasted - Plot Twist

To my surprise, my workouts **did not suffer** – they improved.

No sluggish digestion. No regret mid-burpee.

I was lifting heavier, moving better, and my post-workout protein panic?

Gone. I simply shifted my meal to my eating window.

No muscle loss. Just myth loss.

From 16:8 to OMAD: The Bold Leap

As my body adapted, I experimented with eating windows –

16:8…18:6…20:4… and then came the mighty **OMAD (One Meal A Day).**

At first, OMAD sounded like something monks do before levitating.

But weirdly, it worked.

And Then… COVID Hit (April 2021)

Just as I had found my rhythm with OMAD, life decided to *test* that rhythm.

In April 2021, during the peak of India's brutal second wave – **I was the first in our family to get infected with COVID.**

It felt like the floor dropped beneath me. We lived with both sets of elderly parents – and the guilt hit like a truck.

And within days – my daughter tested positive. Then my mother.

The first 4 days? A blur.

All I did was sleep. My body needed the rest. No strength, no appetite, no energy to even panic.

But once my daughter tested positive, worry set in.

"Who's next?"

The answer – my mom.

The Turning Point: Recovery That Surprised Me

By the time my mom was down, I had already begun recovering – still quarantined but functional.

Here's the thing though:

My recovery was faster than expected.

Why?

Because my body wasn't depleted. I had been taking care of it long before the virus came knocking.

While the world rushed to stock up on Vitamin C and Zinc, I was already on it – and not just the generic kind. I was consuming the bioavailable kind –

meaning:

"nutrients that your body can actually absorb and use, not just flush out."

When I tested negative, I was back on my feet – **driving to INHS Ashwini to see my mom.**

Yes, she got hospitalized – just to be safe.

And I got the rest of the family vaccinated while managing groceries, meds, and care duties.

The Lesson? Health Is Never a One-Time Download

That period taught me two things:

Supplements matter.

So does everything you do BEFORE you fall sick.

Because *that* becomes your body's ammunition during the fight.

Even though the world was in collective panic, even though the stress was high – I wasn't broken.

I bent, yes.

But I didn't break.

And I owe that resilience to:

Intermittent fasting

Nutritional supplementation

and above all... **being in tune with my body.**

One Meal a Day, and a Life That Feels Full

So here I am – the same woman who once panicked at the thought of skipping a meal –

Now thriving on one powerhouse plate a day.

Do I still dream of samosas at 11 AM sometimes?

Absolutely.

But do I wake up feeling powerful, clear-headed, and grateful for the choices I've made?

Every single day.

PART III:

BUILDING A SUSTAINABLE ENERGY SYSTEM

Chapter 7

Time is Your New Superfood

The Science and Simplicity of Fasting for Busy People

If someone had told me 10 years ago that "not eating all the time" would become the next big health trend, I would've laughed – probably while chewing on something.

But here we are.

Fasting has become the new multivitamin – except it's free, has no packaging, and doesn't expire in your kitchen drawer.

And the best part? You don't have to buy anything.

You don't need imported goji berries, fancy smoothies, or a subscription to some almond-milk-delivery startup in Bandra.

All you need… is a clock.

Wait… Not Eating is Good for You?

Sounds counterintuitive, right?

Especially when we've been raised in India on a solid three-meals-a-day (plus snacks, chai breaks, and some emotional eating just to round it off).

But here's the truth:

Our bodies were not designed to eat from the moment we wake up to the moment we sleep.

Back in the day — before Swiggy, Netflix, and fridge raids at 11 PM — we humans had natural fasting windows.

We hunted, gathered, cooked, ate, and then… waited.

There was no midnight dal-chawal.

Our ancestors didn't say, "Let me just open the fridge and find something low-carb."

They had to fast — it was built into survival.

Now?

We "survive" without snacks for two hours and start yelling "low BP lag raha hai!"(feels like I have Low BP)

So, What Exactly Is Intermittent Fasting (IF)?

Let's break it down — simply.

Intermittent Fasting is not a diet.

It doesn't tell you what to eat. It tells you when to eat.

You cycle between periods of eating and periods of not eating — and during that "not eating" phase, your body finally gets to focus on repairing, cleaning, and burning fat instead of constantly digesting idlis and parathas.

Most common format?

16:8 = Fast for 16 hours, eat in an 8-hour window.

So if you have your first meal at 12 PM and last meal at 8 PM – boom! You're fasting till next day noon.

No food. No chai with sugar.

(Yes, black coffee and plain water are allowed. So is nimbu-pani without the sugar drama.)

The Science - But Made Simple

Let's keep it less "Harvard Medical Journal" and more "even-your-chachi-would-understand."

When we eat – especially carbs – our body releases insulin, a hormone that helps store glucose (sugar) from food into cells.

But if insulin is always high (because we're eating all day), our body never gets to burn fat.

Intermittent fasting lowers insulin levels, which signals the body:

"Hey! No food incoming – let's use this stored fat now."

That's fat-burning, detox, and hormone regulation all in one.

Plus, fasting has been shown to:

- [x] Improve digestion
- [x] Reduce inflammation
- [x] Support better blood sugar levels
- [x] Boost brain clarity
- [x] Reduce belly fat (yes, that stubborn pooch!)

But What About My Chai and Biscuits?

Ah yes – the National Combo of India™.

I get it. The emotional connection to chai-biscuit is real.

But when you're constantly breaking your fast with milk tea and glucose biscuits, you're giving your body sugar rollercoasters it never asked for.

Swap it with black coffee, green tea, cinnamon water, or just plain warm water.

You'll be amazed at how much calmer your digestion and mood feel when you're not constantly snacking "just because."

Fasting for Busy Bees (a.k.a You and Me)

You're a professional. A parent. A go-getter. You don't have time to count calories or cook elaborate meals with 14 ingredients.

That's why fasting is perfect for busy people. Here's why:

No meal prep in the morning

Less decision fatigue (What to eat? becomes Not yet.)

You're more alert during work hours (because digestion isn't slowing you down)

You automatically eat fewer calories without trying too hard

And trust me, after a while, your body actually loves this rhythm.

You stop waking up hangry.

Your energy is stable.

You don't crash post lunch.

You stop living from snack to snack like a squirrel in Diwali mode.

But Will I Lose Muscle? Faint? Get Weak?

Let's bust these myths:

No, your body won't eat your muscles.

If you're eating enough protein and nutrients during your eating window – and staying active – you'll retain (or even gain) lean muscle mass.

No, you won't faint.

That's just your old sugar addiction talking. Drink water. Take electrolytes if needed. Breathe.

No, you don't need six meals a day to "boost metabolism."

Desi Tip: Listen to Your Body, Not Your WhatsApp Auntie Group

Everyone's fasting window will look different.

Start slow. Maybe 12:12. Then try 14:10. Then 16:8.

Listen to your body.

Track your energy.

Notice your digestion.

Sleep better. Poop better. Think better.

And if someone asks why you skipped breakfast, tell them:

"I'm not starving, I'm healing."

One Final Note

Food is not the enemy. Time is not the enemy.

Your habits are not broken — they're just... misinformed.

Intermittent fasting helps you bring structure, clarity, and joy back into eating.

It helps your body do what it was designed to do.

You don't need imported supplements.

You need time, trust, and a little turmeric.

"You don't need more willpower. You just need fewer eating windows."

Chapter 8

Structured to Shine

How We Designed Our Day Around Productivity and Recovery

One of the best things that came out of our OMAD journey wasn't just fat loss, better digestion, or glowing skin (although yes, all of that happened – thank you, metabolism!).

It was this unexpected superpower: **time freedom and mental clarity.**

Let's rewind to 2020 – post-lockdown.

While most people were lining up for banana bread and dalgona coffee tutorials, my husband and I were happily continuing our **One Meal A Day** lifestyle.

No, we weren't secretly training for a Himalayan trek.

And no, we weren't saving money on groceries (although, that too, happened).

We just... felt good.

Really good.

By then, our bodies were **so aligned with this new rhythm** that eating less often didn't feel like restriction – it felt like relief.

Designing Our Day (Without a Watch)

Once the world opened up and routines returned, we noticed something beautiful:

We no longer built our day around food.

We built it around purpose.

There was no more:

"Breakfast at 8, snack at 11, lunch by 1, chai at 4, dinner by 8, guilt by 9."

Now, we had **space.** Mental, emotional, digestive space.

We still had our work meetings, client calls, grocery runs, and family stuff – but now, **without the pressure of "what to eat next."**

I Stopped Watching the Clock. I Started Listening to My Body.

This was a big one for me.

In the beginning, I used to obsess over the fasting window:

"Is it 16 hours yet? Can I eat now?"

I had 3 timers and a mental countdown like it was a cricket match.

But over time, I stopped being a slave to the clock.

I tuned into something better – **my own signals.**

Some days, I'd feel genuine hunger earlier than usual – maybe due to an intense workout, PMS or a mentally draining day. So, I ate.

And some days? I was so immersed in my work or feeling so light and focused, I'd hit **20+ hours** without even realizing.

That's when I truly understood freedom from food fixation.

It wasn't about "how long can I fast?"

It was, "how do I feel right now?"

Energy Levels That Shocked Me (in a Good Way)

As a weight loss and gut health coach, my day involves deep conversations – sometimes emotional, sometimes analytical, always energetic.

And here's the wild part:

I was sharper at hour 18 than I ever was after a big breakfast.

There's something magical about fasting and focus.

No post-lunch slump.

No chai-craving drama.

No sugar crashes or brain fog.

Just... clarity.

I could go from a client session to a content strategy call to a full-blown Zoom workshop – without needing a snack to keep me sane.

That, to me, was a bigger win than any jeans size.

How We Structured Our Day (Without Obsessing Over It)

There's no rigid schedule in our house.

We just follow a **loose, flexible rhythm** based on two anchors:

🧠 **Mental sharpness during the day**

🍽 **A nutrient-dense meal when the body says it's time**

A Typical Day in My Fasting Life (Pitta-Friendly, Performance-Ready)

Morning (Fast State):

I start my day with **black coffee** or **warm water**, sometimes infused with a pinch of **rock salt** or **cinnamon** – depending on how my body feels.

Then it's time to move – either **strength training** or **a recovery run** if I've been training for an upcoming marathon.

No breakfast. No panic. Just me, my breath, and a solid playlist.

After that, it's work mode: client consults, strategy planning, content creation — all while fasting and surprisingly focused.

Midday (Eating Window):

By around 1 PM – when **Pitta is at its peak** – I have my **one main meal of the day**.

This is my royal plate:

Balanced, wholesome, high in **clean protein**, good fats like **ghee or coconut oil**, and lots of **veggies** and herbs to support digestion and performance.

No counting calories, no guilt — just **satisfying, soul-nourishing food.**

Evening (Still in the Fast):

I skip dinner.

Yes – on purpose.

Why? Because eating late doesn't suit my body type (hello, Pitta!) or my sleep quality.

And let's be honest – digestion after 8 PM usually feels like a night shift no one signed up for.

Instead, I hydrate, wind down, maybe do a light walk or stretching, and focus on **rest and recovery** – because marathons are won not just in training, but in how well you **rebuild**.

"I don't eat less. I eat once — with intention. And it fuels everything I do."

The Indian Twist: Yes, This Works with Our Food Too

You don't have to give up your rajma-chawal or thepla.

You just need to **time it right** and **balance it well.**

Once a day, we eat like royalty — with real food, made with love (and ghee), minus the noise of six tiny, unsatisfying meals that feel like unscheduled interviews with your stomach.

"Your energy isn't just from what you eat. It's from when you give your body space to thrive."

If you're reading this thinking,

"But I have a 9-to-5 job, client meetings, school runs — how will I manage this?"

I've got you.

In the next chapter, we'll explore **exactly how to transition into this lifestyle — step by step — and make it work even if you have back-to-back calls, a chatty boss, and a kitchen full of temptations**

Chapter 9

Simplify to Satisfy

What I Eat, How I Prepare, and Why Less is Truly More

When people hear "One Meal A Day," their first reaction is usually a dramatic gasp, followed by,

"But what do you even eat?"

Let me assure you: I don't survive on lettuce leaves and hope.

I eat **real food**. I eat **nutritious food**. I eat with joy, intention, and **zero guilt.**

And no — I'm not punishing myself. I'm **fueling** my life, my workouts, my runs, my business, and my purpose.

The Plate That Powers Me

As a nutritionist, I didn't reach this lifestyle through shortcuts or social media trends.

I reached here by doing what I now tell every client:

Listen to your body. It's wiser than any fad.

I took care of my **macros** (protein, fats, carbs) and my **micros** (vitamins, minerals).

I trained hard. I ran my miles. And I noticed how food felt – not just how it tasted.

Today, my one meal is not an emotional buffet.

It's a beautifully balanced, **nourishing experience.**

On a regular day, my lunch looks like this:

Red rice

Homemade dal

One sabzi (whatever's seasonal and colourful)

Curd for gut health

One fruit (sometimes papaya, sometimes apple – never watermelon in winter, okay?)

And guess what?

I feel satisfied.

Light.

Alive.

Not bloated, not sleepy, not scanning the fridge for "something crunchy" an hour later.

Less is More (But Never Less Nutrition)

There's a myth that eating less = being deprived.

Not true.

Eating **right** is about eating what your body needs, not what the clock says or what your emotions crave.

I don't avoid the foods I love.

If I want something, I have it – but **mindfully**.

A few bites of a dessert? Sure.

A piece of chocolate? Absolutely.

But I don't let the treat become a habit or a reward system.

My relationship with food is peaceful, not performative.

The Sunday Chai Ritual

Now let me confess something wild –

I have tea **only once a week**, and that too **on Sundays**.

It's become a small, cozy ritual I look forward to –

Not an addiction, not a crutch, just a mindful moment of joy.

Because when your body is balanced, you don't **need** caffeine to function.

You **choose** it for flavour, for tradition, for comfort.

Please Don't Jump to OMAD – Here's the Real Path

I know OMAD sounds powerful (and it is!), but **please don't jump into it overnight.**

For me, it was a **slow, patient progression** – like building muscle or saving for your dream vacation.

If you're inspired to begin your intermittent fasting journey, here's my advice:

Start with a 12-hour fasting window.

Let's say you finish dinner at 8 PM — don't eat anything until 8 AM.

No midnight snacks. No "just one biscuit." Not even fruit.

Once your body gets used to this, and you can complete it comfortably for 2–3 weeks, **move to 14:10.**

That means fasting for 14 hours, and eating in a 10-hour window.

Stay here for at least **a month**. Let your body adjust. Let your metabolism stabilize.

Then, and only then, try **16:8.**

And if, eventually, your body thrives on OMAD — fantastic.

But if not, that's fine too. Fasting is a **tool**, not a trophy.

"Your body isn't a battleground. It's your lifelong home. Fuel it with respect."

And one more thing —

Always, always consult a qualified professional before making big changes to your eating pattern.

Because your health is personal. And your journey deserves guidance.

Chapter 10
Movement is Medicine

How Running and Strength Training Transformed My Mind and Metabolism

Let me tell you a secret.

Until the age of **36**, I hadn't stepped into a gym.

Why?

Because somewhere deep down, I believed what many women are still told:

"Lifting weights will make you bulky."

I imagined biceps bigger than my handbag and veins popping out while I tried to fry an egg.

So instead, I danced, I did yoga, I walked, I tried Zumba.

All great forms of movement – but still, something was missing.

It wasn't until I understood the **science** that I realized how **wrong** I was – and more importantly, how much **time I had wasted** avoiding the very thing that would take my health to the next level.

The Tripod of True Health

Health isn't built on one magical diet or workout.

It's built on a **tripod**:

Sleep

Nutrition

Strength Training

Miss even one, and you're always playing catch-up.

By the time I finally walked into a gym, I had already spent **six solid months** cleaning up my food, aligning my eating pattern, and getting my sleep in check.

So, when I picked up that first dumbbell?

Boom. Transformation.

Not just physically – but mentally.

My personal trainer was shocked. "You're lifting like you've been training for years!"

But the truth was simple: **My body was already ready.**

Because I'd been feeding it right, sleeping well, and removing all the internal chaos.

The Power of Lifting (Especially for Women)

Let me say this loud and clear:

Strength training is not optional. Especially for women.

It's not just about muscles.

It's about:

- Bone density (bye-bye osteoporosis fears)
- Hormonal balance
- Joint strength
- Metabolic firepower
- Confidence like you've never felt before

I started lifting light. Then slowly progressed.

Deadlifts, squats, kettlebell swings — words that once sounded intimidating became part of my weekly love language.

And guess what?

I didn't bulk up.

I **shaped up**.

I became stronger, leaner, more graceful — in body and mind.

Running for the Soul, Lifting for the Core

Alongside strength training, I ran.

Not to punish my body. But to **celebrate what it could do.**

Running gave me mental stillness.

Strength training gave me physical power.

Together? They built **resilience**.

Now, I look forward to long runs, race days, sweaty lifting sessions, and even the next-day soreness — because all of it reminds me of how far I've come.

What Held Me Back? Me.

Sometimes I wonder:

Why didn't I start earlier?

Who was stopping me?

And the answer is simple (and slightly uncomfortable):

It was me.

My own notions. My fears. My outdated beliefs.

No one told me I couldn't lift weights — I just assumed it wasn't "for me."

I laugh at that version of myself now — and send her love.

Because once I started combining smart nutrition with purposeful movement, it was like finally driving a car with the **handbrake released.**

I wasn't dragging myself anymore.

I was **flowing forward.**

"Movement isn't punishment. It's medicine. And every woman deserves to feel strong — from the inside out."

So, here's my advice:

Don’t wait.

Don’t wait to “lose weight” before you pick up a dumbbell.

Don’t wait to feel ready.

Don’t wait for a perfect time.

Because the **earlier you start**, the stronger your future self will thank you.

PART IV:

LIFESTYLE, MINDSET & ROUTINE

Chapter 11

Sleep, Stress & the Silent Killers

Why Your Pot Belly Isn't About the Paratha

Let's talk about the elephant in the room.

Or more accurately... the **belly fat that refuses to budge**, no matter how clean you eat or how perfectly you portion your meals.

I see this all the time – clients doing everything "right":

☑ Eating homemade meals

☑ Controlling carbs

☑ Watching portions

☑ Drinking enough water

☑ Even whispering motivational quotes to their quinoa bowls

But still...

That pot belly?

Stays like a clingy ex.

So... what's going on?

It's Not the Food, It's the Sleep (or Lack of It)

Let me ask you this:

What happens the minute you hit the bed?

Do you switch off like a yogi in nirvana?

No. You "reward yourself."

Just a little scrolling.

Just one reel.

Maybe one episode. Okay two. Fine, let's just finish the whole series.

And boom – it's midnight.

And your brain is doing cardio, not your body.

In this drama, your **sleep** takes the hit.

And here's the kicker:

If your body doesn't sleep well, it doesn't recover. It doesn't burn fat.

It simply goes into **survival mode**.

And in survival mode, the body says:

"Hmm. We're stressed. Let's store fat – especially in the abdomen. Just in case we need it to fight tigers or deadlines tomorrow."

This is where **cortisol**, the stress hormone, becomes the villain.

Lack of sleep = ↑ Cortisol = ↓ Fat burn = ↑ Belly fat.

So if you're wondering why your tummy won't flatten despite all your food sacrifices – blame your 1 AM binge-watch, not your besan chilla.

Sleep Is Your Fat-Burning Friend

Sleep is when the body:

Repairs muscles

Balances hormones

Regulates hunger signals

Clears mental fog

AND burns fat efficiently

Without sleep, ghrelin (your hunger hormone) gets louder.

Leptin (your fullness hormone) goes missing.

And your willpower? Disappears like your charger when you need it most.

Structure = Sanity (and a Smaller Waist)

Want to change your body?

Start by **training your body to expect a rhythm** – like clockwork.

Let me explain with a simple truth:

When you wake up, do you think about brushing your teeth?

Nope.

You just do it.

It's automatic – a beautiful case of **muscle memory**.

Now imagine if your meals, workouts, and sleep followed that same automation?

That's why I swear by **structure** and **routine**.

You don't have to live like a robot. But your body thrives when it knows what's coming next.

The 90-Minute Rule That Can Change Your Life

Here's my golden rule:

Give your body a 90-minute block to work with.

If you wake up at **6:00 AM on weekdays**, then on weekends, don't sleep beyond **7:30 AM**.

That one-and-a-half-hour cushion gives your body enough flexibility to rest, while still maintaining **circadian rhythm consistency**.

And this applies to all major activities:

Activity	Ideal Range (90-min window)
Wake-up time	6:00 - 7:30 AM
Breakfast	8:00 - 9:30 AM
Lunch	1:00 - 2:30 PM
Dinner	7:00 - 8:30 PM
Sleep time	10:00 - 11:30 PM

The more regularly your body sees this pattern, the **more efficient it becomes at fat burning**, digestion, mood balance, and yes — flattening that stubborn belly.

Track It to Transform It - Your Weekly Rhythm Tracker

Because what gets **measured**, gets **mastered**.

Here's your weekly rhythm activity sheet. Print it. Stick it on your fridge. Use it like a lifestyle mirror:

Day	Wake-Up Time	Breakfast Time	Lunch Time	Dinner Time	Sleep Time
Monday					
Tuesday					
Wednesday					
Thursday					
Friday					
Saturday					
Sunday					

Consistency isn't boring. It's powerful.

And your body absolutely loves it.

Chapter 12
Nutrition Beyond Fads

Gut Health, Whole Foods & Food Freedom

If I had a coin for every time a client walked in saying,

"I saw this new diet trend on Instagram, can I try it?"

...I could buy enough chia seeds to fill an Olympic pool.

One of my clients, who joined my **year-long program**, would turn up every month with a new fad diet request – carnivore one month, fruit-only the next, and at one point, something called the "no water till 6 PM" challenge. I had to gently remind him:

"You signed up for a transformation. Not a tasting menu of nutrition trends."

I don't do monthly plans – because the body doesn't work on a 30-day billing cycle.

It works with **consistency, patience, and nourishment** – not new diets every full moon.

Let's Talk Goals (The Real Ones)

Before you jump onto any diet or detox you saw on someone's highlight reel, ask yourself:

"What is my health goal?"

Here's your space. Be honest:

📝 **Write Your Top 5 Health Goals:**

____

____

____

____

____

Now look at your list.

Did you write "I want to look like a model"?

If yes – totally fine. No judgement. We all want to feel good in our jeans.

But did you also write things like:

"Improve energy levels"

"Get rid of bloating or inflammation"

"Be able to play a sport or run 5K"

"Lift a certain weight"

That's what I call **real goals**.

Because here's the truth:

When your insides are healthy, the outside naturally reflects it.

Start From Within: Why You Need to Detox

Before you get on another "clean eating" plan –

you need to **clear the toxins** that are already sitting in your gut like unwelcome relatives.

How do these toxins build up?

Overeating processed food

Too much sugar or alcohol

Antibiotics and poor digestion

Lack of fiber

Sleep deprivation

Constant stress

And when your gut is overloaded, your **liver takes the hit.**

A **fatty liver** doesn't just affect digestion – it slows down **fat metabolism, energy levels, and hormonal function.**

Imagine asking a tired employee to do 10 people's jobs. That's your liver when it's inflamed.

Detox Is Not a Trend – It's Ancient Wisdom

Every culture has detox built into it:

Hindus – Navratri & weekly fasting

Muslims – Ramzan (month-long intermittent fasting!)

Christians – Lent

Jains – Annual fasting rituals

This wasn't just about faith – it was biology.

Our ancestors were giving their bodies a **reset button**.

So yes, even today – detoxing once every 3-4 months is a gift to your gut and liver.

And no – detox doesn't mean juice cleanse. It means real food, real rest, real rhythm.

The Fasting FAQ Everyone Asks:

"What Can I Eat During a Fast?"

It's not about what to eat, it's about what not to eat.

Start with:

Water

Herbal teas

Lime water without sugar

Coconut water (in moderation)

Light fruits or broth-based soups, if needed

Once this **cleansing process** is complete, move into the phase of **whole food eating** – where most of your plate is homemade, unprocessed, and close to nature.

Measure What Matters: Fat Loss, Not Just Weight Loss

Here's a fact I wish more people knew:

Your body weight includes bones, muscles, fat, organs, and fluids.

So, stop obsessing over the number on the scale.

Start tracking **inches.**

Because **inch loss = fat loss**, and fat loss = better metabolism, energy, and long-term health.

3-Month Action Plan

Do a proper detox (with support)

Eat whole, homemade food

Follow a structured routine

Track your inch loss – not just kilos

Your Personal Measurement Tracker

Fill it once a month. Let your results speak – not the scale.

Date	Weight (kg)	Chest (cm)	Waist (cm)	Abdomen (cm)	Hips (cm)	Arms (R)	Arms (L)	Thighs (R)	Thighs (L)	Calf (R)	Calf (L)

"Stop chasing perfection. Start chasing progress – inside out."

Chapter 13

Social Life, Travel & Real-Life Adaptation

Saying No Without Guilt and Staying Consistent on the Go

Let's talk about one of life's greatest joys: **vacations.**

And one of health's biggest curveballs: **vacation food.**

Now I travel 4–5 times a year (yes, I love it!) – and between beach trips, hill holidays, weddings, and business travels, one thing became clear:

It's not travel that breaks your routine.

It's what you **tell yourself** while travelling.

Like:

"It's okay, I'm on a break."

"I'll start clean after this trip."

"Just one more croissant can't hurt…"

And my personal favourite:

"I paid for the buffet. I MUST do justice."

Buffets: Where Hunger Meets Hysteria

Let's address the morning buffet situation.

You walk in fresh and determined…

…only to spot live counters, 4 varieties of cheese, 3 types of breads, a dosa station, and 9 colourful juices (all labelled "fresh").

Suddenly you think:

"I deserve all of this. I'm on vacation!"

So what do you do?

You get everything.

A bit of upma, one pancake, 2 boiled eggs, 3 pieces of fruit, one random Danish, and a croissant – just to balance things out.

Then you sit down, eat it all, and… don't even remember what tasted good.

Here's the truth:

Your body doesn't know you paid ₹1200 for that breakfast.

It only knows how much it has to **digest**.

The Better Way to Do Buffets (Without Being a Bore)

Step 1: Walk around. Yes, walk.

Look at what's available before you pick up the plate like it's Diwali sale at a sari store.

Step 2: Take what your body needs **first** – protein, some healthy fats, veggies if available, and a small carb.

Eat it. Chew it. Breathe.

Step 3: After 10 minutes, pause and ask:

"Am I still hungry or just excited by variety?"

Step 4: If you truly feel the need, go back for one more small plate.

You'll still enjoy your food, but you'll do it mindfully – and your gut will thank you.

Business Travel, Not a Free Pass

Business trips are usually packed with meetings, long days, airport stress, and hotel buffets that seem like the only reward.

But remember this – **you don't owe anyone poor eating habits just because you're not home.**

I follow 3 simple things while travelling for work:

Stay hydrated. Airports and flights are dehydrating – drink water every chance you get.

Stick to 2 meals. With less movement, fewer meals work better.

Protein first, taste later. At every meal, I scan the options and lock in protein first – eggs, paneer, chicken, dal, chana. Then I add the "fun stuff."

No guilt, no panic. Just awareness.

Saying No (Without Sounding Like a Party Pooper)

You don't need to carry a Tupperware to social dinners (unless it's a potluck!).

You also don't need to give long speeches about your eating routine.

A polite:

"I'm full, thank you."

or

"That looks lovely, but I'll skip the dessert today."

is more than enough.

The people who truly matter won't force you to eat.

And the ones who do? Probably need this book more than you do 😉

To-Do List: Eating Out Without Losing Your Balance

To Do
Look at the full menu before ordering.
Eat slowly, chew well.
Prioritize protein and fiber-rich foods.
Stop eating when you're 80% full.
Drink water throughout.
Plan one indulgence, not ten.
Enjoy conversations more than courses.
Say no politely – guilt-free.

Not-To-Do List: Common Pitfalls While Eating Out

Not To Do
Don't land up starving – you'll overeat.
Don't say "I'll make up for it tomorrow."
Don't justify overeating with "YOLO."
Don't skip meals before to "compensate."
Don't mix too many cuisines in one meal.
Don't eat just because it's on your plate.
Don't apologize for choosing health.

"Travelling and dining out are part of life – not reasons to abandon the life you're building."

PART V:

THE COACH IN ME

Chapter 14

Helping Others Heal

From Personal Journey to Purposeful Coaching

When people ask me how I became a coach, I tell them the truth:

I didn't choose this path. This path chose me — through my own transformation.

For years, I struggled with the same things many of my clients do today:

Fluctuating energy, belly fat that wouldn't budge, bloating, inflammation, and that feeling of being disconnected from my own body.

I was juggling family, work, social life — and still putting myself last.

But slowly, through food, movement, fasting, and deeper awareness... I came back home — to me.

And I didn't walk this path alone.

Transformation Begins at Home: Our Journey

My husband and I took this journey together.

We questioned what we were taught about health.

We gave up midnight snacking and embraced time-restricted eating.

We went from sugar crashes to stable energy, from skipping workouts to strength training and marathons.

Together, we rewrote our relationship with food, sleep, movement - and most importantly, with **discipline**.

We weren't aiming for abs or Insta-worthy plates.

We were aiming for **freedom** - from brain fog, fatigue, disease, and guesswork.

And when I saw how this lifestyle changed us -not just physically, but emotionally and mentally - I knew I couldn't keep it to myself.

From Nutritionist to Coach – The Shift

When I first started, I worked as a **nutrition consultant** — offering personalized 1:1 plans to clients.

Yes, they got results.

But something felt incomplete.

Because transformation isn't about handing someone a PDF and hoping they follow it.

It's about holding space.

Asking better questions.

Helping them remember their "why" when motivation disappears.

That's when I stepped into **coaching.**

As a coach, I don't just focus on what you eat.

I focus on why you eat.

When you eat.

How you feel before and after.

What is getting in the way — in your mind, routine, and energy.

It's Not Just About Food — It's About Focus

In my coaching, I combine:

Mindset alignment

Somatic tools like breathwork, tapping, journaling

Structured rituals to build discipline

And yes — a solid nutrition and fasting protocol

Because let's be honest — life will always be busy.

But when you learn to tune in, get intentional, and make space for your why, your body listens. And it responds.

Your WHY is Your Anchor

You can have the best meal plan in the world.

But if you don't have a reason that fuels you **every single day**, it won't last.

That's why in my coaching program's, I always begin with this:

"Why do you want to transform?"

Not the surface answer.

Not just "I want to lose weight."

But the deeper reason.

To feel alive again.

To run with your kids.

To stop depending on medications.

To glow from the inside.

To enter your 40s, 50s and beyond **stronger** -not sicker.

2000+ Lives. One Mission.

Today, I've had the honor of coaching over **2000 individuals** – each with their own story, struggle, and spark.

From busy professionals to leaders, and retirees – I've helped them **reclaim their health** and finally build habits that stick.

Not through just 30-day challenges.

Not through guilt or extreme diets.

But through understanding.

Through simplicity.

Through compassionate coaching.

"Healing isn't a quick fix. It's a lifelong friendship with your body."

And now, dear reader - it's your turn.

You've read my journey.

You've reflected on your own.

Now it's time to ask:

What is your WHY?

Write it down. Stick it on your mirror. Read it every day.

Because when you're tired, tempted, or distracted – your WHY will be your lighthouse.

Final Chapter: Your Reset Starter Kit

Bonus Toolkit & Action Steps

You've read the journey.

You've laughed, reflected, scribbled in margins (I hope), and maybe even paused to sip some jeera water.

Now comes the most important part –

Putting it into action.

Because transformation doesn't come from information.

It comes from **application.**

So here's your **starter toolkit** – everything you need to begin your own journey toward vibrant health, clear energy, and long-term freedom.

Meal Plan Template for 16:8 (Vegetarian & Balanced)

This plan assumes your **eating window is from 12 PM to 8 PM.**

Time	Meal Description
12:00 PM	**Lunch (Main Meal)** 1 cup red rice or millet roti Cooked sabzi with ghee 1 bowl dal (moong/masoor/toor) Paneer bhurji / chana salad / Salad (cucumber, tomato, beet, lemon) 1 small bowl curd 1 seasonal fruit
4:00 PM	**Snack** Handful of makhana roasted in ghee OR Coconut pieces with soaked almonds & walnuts OR Green tea / infused water
7:30 PM	**Light Dinner (optional on some days)** Veg soup with lentils or moong sprouts Steamed veg + sauteed paneer cubes

Focus: Balanced macros, 1st class vegetarian protein (paneer, legumes), good fats, fiber, hydration

Avoid: Bread, maida-based snacks, packaged juices, late-night sweet cravings

Non-Veg Balanced 16:8 Meal Plan

Eating Window: 12 PM - 8 PM

Time	Time Meal Description
	1 cup red rice OR 2 millet rotis
	Cooked seasonal sabzi with 1 tsp ghee
	1 bowl dal (moong/masoor/toor)

Non-veg protein option: grilled chicken breast (100–120g) OR fish (pomfret, rohu, basa, or salmon - 120g) OR boiled eggs (2 whole + 1 white)

Fresh salad: cucumber, tomato, beetroot, lemon dressing

1 small bowl curd (plain, unsweetened)

1 seasonal fruit (guava, apple, berries, papaya) |

4:00 PM - Snack - Handful of roasted makhana in ghee OR

1 boiled egg + coconut slices OR

Soaked almonds & walnuts with green tea / infused water

7:30 PM - Light Dinner *(optional on some days)* - Clear chicken soup OR fish broth with vegetables + lentils OR

Steamed vegetables with 1 boiled egg or shredded chicken (80–100g) sautéed in olive oil or ghee

Sprinkle fresh herbs and black pepper for flavour |

Focus Points:

Balanced macros - Lean animal protein + plant-based sources for fiber and micronutrients

Healthy fats - Ghee, coconut, nuts, seeds, fatty fish

Hydration - Minimum 2.5–3 L water/infused water daily

Protein priority - Every meal includes a quality protein source

Avoid - Fried meats, processed meats (sausages, salami), maida-based snacks, packaged juices, sugary sauces

Weekly Progress Tracker

Use this to monitor your habits — not just your weight.

Day	Wake-up	Water Intake (L)	Movement (Y/N)	Fasting Window (hrs)	Mood	Energy (1–5)	Bloating (Y/N)
Monday							
Tuesday							
Wednesday							
Thursday							
Friday							
Saturday							
Sunday							

Mindset Journal Prompts

These daily prompts will help anchor your WHY and keep your transformation mental and physical:

Why did I start this journey?

How did I treat my body today – with love or obligation?

Where did I feel the strongest today – mentally or physically?

What's one small win I can celebrate right now?

What would the healthiest version of me do in this situation?

Write just 3-5 lines per day. You'll be amazed how mindset shifts become identity shifts.

Client Case Studies & Testimonials

1. My Transformation Journey - From a Sedentary Lockdown to Running Strong Again

Hi, I'm **Mahesh Kelkar**, a Chartered Accountant by profession. I've always been a studious individual since school and never really engaged in sports. It wasn't until 2017 when a friend introduced me to the world of running that things began to shift. I started participating in 10Ks and half marathons, running 2-3 times a week, with my long runs on Sundays.

But then came **Covid**.

The lockdown disrupted everything. I stopped running completely, and my eating habits took a nosedive. I was constantly snacking on chips, ice cream, and high-calorie, high-sodium junk. My weight shot up from **66 kg to 85 kg**, and my blood reports showed early signs of pre-diabetes. That was a wake-up call.

Determined to take control, I got back into fitness – resumed running on Sundays and joined a gym. But despite my efforts, I wasn't seeing the right results. Without proper nutritional guidance, I was losing weight, yes, but also **losing muscle**. I looked leaner, but not healthier or stronger. People noticed the weight loss, but I didn't feel or look fit.

Then, in **December 2024**, I came to know about **Anupama**, a nutritionist. We both participated in a marathon event in **February 2025**, and I observed her running **effortlessly**, even surpassing me. That's when I realized: fitness isn't just about running or lifting weights – **nutrition is thc foundation**.

I decided to consult her. She took the time to deeply understand my lifestyle, workout routine, and eating habits. Then she crafted a **personalized and practical diet plan** for me. Just after a **month**, I started noticing positive changes – better energy, improved stamina, and muscle retention. She kept modifying the plan based on my progress.

After **3 months**, the transformation has been incredible:

Weekly running mileage has increased to **25–30 km**

Visible **muscle gain and definition**

Even my **abs have started to show**

From struggling to do 10 burpees, I can now smash **100 burpees in 5 minutes**

All of this was possible **only because of the right nutrition** - and Anupama's guidance. Her plan didn't just help me get back in shape, but it taught me how to **fuel my body the right way**.

I'm truly grateful to her and look forward to continuing this journey. The magic lies in the **right balance** - of diet, exercise, and mindset.

Mahesh Kelkar

2. My Health Journey – From High BP & Weight Gain to Strength & Stamina

Hi, I'm **Priyanka Kelkar**, an MBA in Finance by profession. Honestly, I was never inclined towards fitness. But everything changed during and after my pregnancy – my weight shot up to **72 kg**, and I was diagnosed with **high blood pressure**. I was prescribed a **50 mg BP tablet**, which I continued for almost two years.

Eventually, I realized that **relying on medication long-term** wasn't the solution. I became concerned about its **impact on my kidneys and overall health** in the future. That's when I decided to make a **lifestyle change** and joined a gym.

Despite being regular with **gym workouts and functional training**, I wasn't seeing the results I expected. My **weight wasn't reducing**, and more importantly, my **BP wasn't improving**.

In **February 2025**, I went for my annual health check-up, and the reports weren't encouraging – several parameters were in the red. That was my turning point. I realized **diet** was the missing piece.

That's when I approached **Anupama**, a nutritionist. She took the time to understand **my lifestyle, exercise routine, eating habits**, and health history. Based on that, she created a **personalized, practical diet plan** – nothing extreme, just sustainable and balanced.

Within **just a month**, I started noticing:

Higher energy levels

Improved stamina

Better mood and focus

She continued tweaking the plan based on my progress. Around the same time, I consulted another physician who advised me to **monitor my BP regularly** and suggested that I could start **tapering off the medication**.

Before starting the diet, my weight was **61 kg**. Within **3 months**, I dropped to **54 kg** – and most importantly, I was able to **stop my BP medication** entirely.

That's not all:

I now **lift heavy weights confidently**

My **running endurance** has significantly improved

I feel more **energetic throughout the day**

My **sleep quality** has improved too

This has been a life-changing transformation, not just physically but mentally and emotionally. I'm **truly grateful** to Anupama for guiding me with the right nutrition, and I'm excited to keep progressing on this journey toward better health.

Priyanka Kelkar

3. From Lung Surgery to Marathons: How I Rebuilt My Strength, One Step at a Time

Parmila Sharma a Physiotherapist, entrepreneur, mother, and someone who has discovered strength through struggles and fitness.

My fitness journey started in 2011 after the birth of my son. Like many new mothers, I wanted to regain my health, but with work, family, and constant travel, fitness slowly slipped away.

In 2016, I restarted. I began with 3 km runs and some weight training. One fine day, when the treadmill wasn't available, I stepped outside for a run and that changed everything. I loved the freedom of the road, and soon I signed up for my first 10K. That sense of achievement became addictive, and from there, I moved to 21K and full marathons.

But life tested me. In May 2018, I was diagnosed with tuberculosis, and in March 2019, I underwent lung surgery. It was the lowest phase of my life even simple breathing and walking felt difficult. But I refused to give up. Step by step, I restarted, and over time I came back stronger and more determined. My journey took me to international finish lines like the Amsterdam and Chicago Marathons, which felt like miracles after my surgery.

Alongside this, I also built my professional career founding Krsna's Physio Plus in 2012, leading physiotherapy departments in 8 Paras hospitals, and later establishing Vee Care Clinics to bring holistic healthcare closer to people.

Yet, despite all my efforts, I struggled with weight loss and strength balance. I was running and training, but my body wasn't responding the way I wanted. Then came a turning point while returning from a Mumbai Half Marathon, a fellow runner introduced me to Anupama, a nutritionist. Watching her run so effortlessly inspired me to consult her.

That decision changed everything. She studied my lifestyle, work stress, and training routine, and created a personalized nutrition plan. She corrected my portion sizes, adjusted my protein intake, and balanced my carbs in a way that fueled both recovery and performance. The results were visible within weeks my stamina improved, my recovery became faster, and I began to see muscle retention, definition, and real strength.

I am living proof that setbacks whether illness, surgery, or personal struggles don't end our stories; they prepare us for even greater comebacks. With the right balance of fitness, nutrition, and mindset, transformation isn't just possible it's unstoppable. Today, as I train for triathlons while balancing work, family, and health, I carry this belief with me: every challenge only makes me stronger, sharper, and more determined to keep moving forward.

Parmila Sharma

4. Breaking the Cycle: Overcoming Acidity and Finding Balance

Hi, I'm Arun,

While working at Unimoni Exchange in Oman during Covid, my life turned upside down. My work hours stretched from 7 in the morning till 6 in the evening, leaving me drained. In the rush, I began skipping breakfast, surviving on just a cup of tea. What started as a habit soon became a struggle – within months I was battling severe heartburn and acidity that would flare up so badly, I couldn't eat anything at times.

I consulted doctors and tried medications, but the relief was always temporary. The acidity kept coming back more often, and along with it came unintentional weight loss and constant weakness. It was affecting my energy, focus at work, and even simple daily routines.

That's when my wife suggested I approach Anupama, my cousin and a nutritionist. I shared my lifestyle, eating habits, and medical history with her. She created a personalized diet plan that was realistic for me to follow despite my hectic work schedule.

Within a few months, I noticed the difference – the frequency of acidity reduced drastically, my digestion improved, and I slowly started regaining healthy weight and energy. For the first time in years, I felt like I was in control of my health again.

This turnaround was only possible because of Anupama's guidance, and I will always be grateful to her for helping me get my life back.

Arun Lal

5. From Postpartum Struggle to Strength: Reclaiming My Health and Joy

After my pregnancy, my weight climbed to 68 kgs, and life felt heavier in more ways than one. Simple daily chores became difficult, and with a baby to care for in a foreign land, even the smallest tasks felt overwhelming. To make things worse, I was diagnosed with a disc bulge in my neck and lower back, which meant I couldn't go to the gym or do any form of exercise.

I tried controlling my food intake, hoping it would help, but nothing changed. I felt stuck in a body that wasn't letting me live fully or enjoy motherhood the way I had imagined. That's when I realized I needed help – and I turned to my cousin, Anupama.

I shared my lifestyle, eating habits, and medical history with her. She designed a simple, practical diet plan tailored to my situation – one that I could easily prepare amidst my responsibilities. Slowly, I began noticing a difference: the weight started coming off, my energy levels improved, and I felt lighter both physically and emotionally.

In just six months, I reached my pre-pregnancy weight of 56 kgs – something I never believed was possible. More importantly, I could finally keep up with my little one and manage my daily life without constant exhaustion.

This transformation wouldn't have been possible without Anupama's guidance. I'll always be grateful for how she helped me find myself again.

Athira

6. The Hourglass

When I first turned the hourglass over, I wasn't sure what I was waiting for. Would anything even happen? Would the sand just get stuck? But I kept watching, kept choosing, kept waiting. And then one day, I looked back and realized the hourglass was nearly empty — and so was the version of me I thought would always be there.

Being twelve, turning the hourglass over was not something I could have done alone. My help came in the form of my mother's friend, Miss Anupama, who changed my life in ways I never imagined. Today, I stand closer to the person I always wanted to be. She didn't shrink my plate; she made it smarter. As a child, restrictions were rarely enjoyable — being told "no" to my favorite foods felt unfair, even impossible at times. But when change is truly needed, sacrifice stops feeling like punishment and begins to feel like transformation.

Soon, the invisible changes became impossible to ignore. I watched the number on the scale fall from 69 to 55, and with every drop, my confidence grew. Exercise, however, was never easy for me. In the beginning, I avoided it whenever I could, but Miss Anupama kept pushing me, reminding me that food alone wouldn't complete the journey. Slowly, I gave in. What started as hesitation turned into effort, and I found myself doing around thirty minutes of cardio nearly five days a week. It was hard, and many days I wanted to quit, but the results kept me going. The mirror reflected the difference, my clothes told the story, and soon, so did the people around me. Friends, family, even teachers began to notice. Their words of encouragement became fuel, and for the first time, I realized that the discipline I was building at twelve was shaping not just my body, but the way I saw myself.

At the start of COVID, I was a very chubby kid, and that was the image everyone carried of me throughout online school. So when offline classes finally resumed at the end of seventh grade, that's the version of me my classmates expected to see walk through the doors. But instead, they were met with someone entirely different. A few of them didn't even recognize me at first, and the looks of surprise on their faces were unforgettable. It was like I had pulled off the biggest glow-up in school history, and honestly, it felt pretty good to watch everyone's jaws drop. After that day, I didn't mind answering to "Wait…is that really you?" and "How did you do it?" at least ten times a week.

Everyone in my family played a part in this journey. My mom introduced me to Miss Anupama and, along with our cook, made sure I had three proper meals every single day during the diet. Both of them took extra care to prepare food I would enjoy, while still keeping everything exactly as planned. And believe me, Miss Anupama never made me live on plain, boiled vegetables; she gave me choices that were not only healthy but actually delicious. My dad also played a key role, constantly pushing me on the tough days and reminding me why I had started. And as for Miss Anupama, I owe her more than a thank-you – she wasn't just my nutritionist, she was like the secret ingredient in the recipe of my transformation.

Most of my meals came from the same set of ingredients, and after a while, it did feel monotonous – but I pushed through. The recipes continued to evolve just enough to keep things interesting, and in the early days, Miss Anupama even allowed me to snack occasionally and took it easy on me, which made the whole process feel far less daunting. This diet never truly felt like a punishment; it was more like having a supportive friend walking beside me, guiding me and reminding me why I had started. On the toughest days, when I felt like giving up, I would catch my reflection in the mirror and think: there's no turning back now. Too much time, effort, and hope had already been invested in creating this new version of myself.

And whenever I glanced backward, I could only see the old me – a version I could no longer tolerate. Quitting wasn't an option; after all, I had survived math homework, online classes, and a million Zoom freezes. Giving up on myself now would have been like trying to bail out of a rollercoaster mid-loop – and I wasn't about to do that.

Looking back, it feels like I turned an hourglass that was far too heavy for a twelve-year-old to lift – but I never lifted it alone. With Miss Anupama's guidance, my family's constant support, and my own determination, the grains of sand kept slowly falling, reshaping me day by day. The six months that once felt endless now feel like a blink, yet they changed everything. And if you ask me today what I learned, it's this: sometimes the smallest grains of effort create the biggest difference. Also, I learned that an hourglass looks much better when you start to look like one yourself.

Samiksha Manoj

7. From Diabetes & Cholesterol Struggles to a Healthier Lifestyle - How Anupama Changed My Life

I've had the privilege of knowing Anupama for over 15 years—first as a colleague, later as a close friend, and now as someone whose expertise has deeply shaped my life. Back in 2011-12, we were both part of the corporate world. But while most of us stayed, Anupama had the courage to follow her passion. She left the routine behind, embarked on her own fitness journey, and eventually made it her career. Today, she has guided and transformed the lives of many people, myself included.

Although I was always active with running and other workouts, my eating habits reflected a typical corporate lifestyle—irregular, sedentary, and careless. Over time, this led to serious health issues, including diabetes, cholesterol, and uric acid complications. It was during a heartfelt conversation with Anupama that things shifted for me. She reassured me with one simple truth: "Food can correct everything, if you make the right choices."

Her approach is not about crash diets or temporary fixes. She gave me a plan that was realistic, sustainable, and easy to follow. More than just a diet, it was a mindset shift—teaching me how to choose better, manage cravings, and adopt habits I could carry for life. What makes Anupama stand out is her constant engagement—she regularly takes feedback, hosts live seminars and online classes, and even organizes fitness challenges during festivals like Navaratri. These touchpoints keep people like me motivated and ensure we stay on track without derailing.

For me, Anupama is more than a nutritionist. She is a guide, a motivator, and a friend who genuinely cares about helping people live healthier, happier lives.

Vinoth Selvarajan

8. Age Is Just a Number: How I Shed Weight and Regained Health at 78

It was during the Corona period, I used to stay in Mumbai and was almost confined within the four walls of our house owing to the spread of the fatal disease. By then I had already gained a lots of of weight which was 78 kg when I was about 78 years old. I became much concerned about my increasing weight at that age and it was not possible to go out even for walking due to restrictions imposed. At this juncture I came in contact with Mrs Anupama K. Nair, a very renowned Dietician and health adviser. She was very kind enough to give a patient hearing to my submissions and agreed to suggest me necessary exercises and prepared a balanced diet chart for me.

There were also reasons to balance the measurements such as chest, belly, thighs, wrists and ankles. So, she had suggested to me the right diets and exercises as a result of which I could achieve the target and my weight got reduced by 8 kg to 70 kg within a span of 6 months.

I am really grateful to Anupama K. Nair for showing me the right directions and guiding me from time to time enabling me to overcome the situation in respect of my health.

Santimay Kar

9. A Journey of Discipline and Transformation

The transformation journey with my daughter, Anupama – my strict caregiver and now my mentor – has been one of the most remarkable experiences of my life.

Six years ago, my lifestyle looked very different. I never had a proper diet schedule or eating pattern. Food meant convenience, not nourishment. Any kind of food, at any time of the day, seemed acceptable. Fried snacks like nuts and chips were my regular companions, and slowly, they began to take a toll on my health. My cholesterol levels shot up, my energy levels went down, and I constantly felt heavy, tired, and weighed down.

I didn't realize how much damage this unplanned routine was doing until Anupama stepped in. She carefully studied my habits and health reports and then started to guide me with a structured eating pattern. She taught me what to eat, when to eat, and how much to eat. For me, the biggest shift wasn't just in the food, but in the discipline, she encouraged me to build. It wasn't an easy journey at first. Saying no to my favorite fried foods or pushing away a plate of something tasty right in front of me required willpower I didn't know I had. But slowly, as I followed her regime, I began to notice changes.

Now, I can easily go without food for long hours without feeling uncomfortable. Even when tempting, delicious food is placed before me, I don't feel the same urge to eat it – and that's the biggest sign of my transformation.

Today, I feel light, energetic, and empowered. My cholesterol levels are back within the normal range, and I can walk for more than an hour without fatigue — something I would have never imagined earlier.

Perhaps the proudest moment in my journey has been running (Walk & Jog) three marathons in my 70s. They may have been 5 km runs, but for someone who would have laughed at the idea of running a marathon in their 60s, standing at the finish line was a moment of triumph and gratitude.

At 73, I realize that discipline, consistency, and the right guidance can rewrite your story at any age. Anupama not only helped me reset my health but also gave me the confidence to push limits I never thought possible. She has truly been a strong pillar in my life — a caregiver, a mentor, and the reason I now walk (and run) with pride.

Maj Gen (Retd) A Kamalam

10. Unlearning to Relearn: My Transformation Through Nutrition

Anupama has deep knowledge and a detailed approach which brought out the desired weight loss response in my body. She helped me with eliminating decades long errors in my eating choices. She helped me properly time my supplements. She helped me with approaches which helped me replace night time hunger pangs with healthier options. I wish her the very best for her future endeavours.

Amit Pathak

11. When the Gut Heals, Everything Changes

I approached Anu at a time when I had gut issues that was indirectly affecting my mood and overall well-being.

Beyond her superbly curated diet plan, it was her unwavering support, guidance and compassion that healed me and my gut. She stood by me through detox, doubt and discovery - guiding me with patience, uncovering a healthier, balanced version of myself.

ARCHANA MILLU

12. This Time, It Wasn't About Losing Weight—It Was About Finding Myself

For as long as I can remember, my battle wasn't just with food—it was with the mirror, the weighing scale, and my own reflection. Growing up, I was often told a dress or outfit would look better on a 'thinner person.' Those words shaped a bitter relationship with my body and left me believing my worth was tied to the kilos I carried.

I've lost and gained the same weight countless times. But this time, everything changed when I crossed paths with Anupama at the gym. It felt like the universe had sent me a sign that my journey could be different. She showed me that eating healthy doesn't have to mean following a restrictive or fancy diet—it can simply be about small, consistent changes in daily meals and lifestyle.

For the first time, I understood that sustainable weight loss isn't about crash diets or punishments—it's about mindset, habits, patience, and showing up for yourself. Anupama reminded me that falling off the wagon isn't failure if you're willing to climb back on. That truth has stayed with me.

Now, exercise feels like a celebration of what my body can do rather than a punishment for what it isn't. The pride of finishing a workout I almost skipped, the joy of clothes fitting better, and the surge of energy in my daily life—these are victories no scale can measure.

Of course, I still have tough days. There are moments when giving up seems easier, when comfort food calls my name. But I've made up my mind to keep trying, keep showing up, and keep moving forward. This journey is no longer about quick fixes—it's about honoring my body, reclaiming my strength, and believing that I am worth the effort.

Thank you, Anupama, for helping me realize that true transformation isn't a three-month crash course—it's a lifelong journey of health and strength.

Aishwarya Hariharan

13. Fuel for the Finish Line: How Nutrition Transformed My Run

When I resumed marathon training after a long gap, I believed that running more and hitting the gym would be enough to get me back to the track. However, despite my efforts, the results were not great. It became clear that something crucial was missing.

That's when I turned to Anupama for nutritional guidance. Her approach was not about quick fixes or restrictive diets – it was about understanding my training routine, lifestyle, eating habits, and goals, and then crafting a plan that fueled my performance. Within weeks, I felt the difference - my endurance increased, and I could train at a better level.

Today, I'm running stronger, recovering faster, and performing better than ever – all thanks to the right nutrition strategy of Anupama. Kudos to her for transforming my lifestyle.

Lovejeet Singh,

Corporate & Aviation Lawyer

14. My Transformation Journey – A Soldier's Path to Peak Fitness

Hi, I'm Colonel Vinod, having served in the Indian Army. Discipline and fitness have always been integral to my life. Being in the forces, physical training and endurance were part of my daily routine. However, over the years, despite regular workouts and my gym routine, I felt I wasn't getting the kind of results I wanted. My strength was there, but I often felt fatigued, my recovery was slow, and my overall energy levels were not at their best.

That's when I consulted Anupama, a nutritionist whose approach to diet and fitness completely changed the game for me. She carefully studied my lifestyle, my Army schedule, workout patterns, and eating habits before designing a personalized nutrition plan. What impressed me the most was how practical and sustainable her plan was — no crash diets, no extreme restrictions, just smart, balanced, and wholesome nutrition.

Within a few weeks of following her plan, I noticed major improvements — my stamina shot up, recovery time reduced drastically, and I began to feel lighter yet stronger. My performance in the gym improved significantly, and even my Army fitness drills started feeling easier. My sleep quality improved, my digestion became better, and I felt energetic throughout the day.

After a few months, the results have been remarkable:

- Noticeable muscle gain with better definition

- Body fat percentage reduced while retaining lean muscle

- Stamina levels enhanced - now I can push harder in both cardio and strength training

- Improved recovery and reduced fatigue

- Better focus and sharper mental clarity

One of the proudest moments in my journey has been competing in the international bodybuilding competition "Muscle Mania," where I bagged the title of Best Physique in my category. This achievement would not have been possible without the right guidance and nutrition support.

The best part is that I now feel fitter, stronger, and more confident not just as an Army officer but also in my personal life. Anupama's nutrition guidance has truly been a turning point in my fitness journey. Her balanced approach has made me realize that nutrition is the backbone of true strength.

I'm deeply grateful to her for this transformation and highly recommend her expertise to anyone who wishes to take their fitness to the next level.

Col Vinod

15. The Power of Consistency: How I Found Strength, Clarity, and Balance

Being healthy in today's world is often associated with looking fit. However, true health is not just about a lean or muscular body – it is about overall well-being, both physical and emotional. I consider myself fortunate to be in a profession where physical fitness is an essential criterion for growth and performance. Yet, like many, there have been phases of prolonged neglect followed by sudden bursts of effort to "get back in shape," often leaving me feeling drained and unbalanced.

It was during one such period that I turned to my sister, Anupama Nair, whose approach to wellness completely changed my perspective on fitness.

Why Anupama's Program Worked for Me

Anupama's program was truly tailor-made. She carefully considered my dietary preferences, professional demands, frequent postings to remote areas, and the irregular meal timings that come with a demanding professional life. What stood out most was her diligence – she meticulously went through my health reports, lifestyle details, and even food accessibility before designing a plan that was not only effective but sustainable.

The Transformation

The initial days were undoubtedly challenging, but her constant monitoring, guidance, and motivation kept me going. Within weeks, the results were visible – not just on the weighing scale but in my energy levels and overall sense of well-being. I often recall the saying: *"You can lead a horse to water, but you can't make it drink."* Anupama led me to the right path, but it was her faith in me and her unwavering support that made me want to drink – to truly embrace health.

Since then, I've stayed in continuous touch with my mentor, who has guided me toward a state of balance – physically strong, mentally calm, and emotionally grounded. Her program didn't just help me lose weight; it helped me gain clarity, discipline, and vitality.

One day, I half-jokingly asked her, "Isn't it a loss of revenue for you once your clients follow your program and no longer need you?"

She smiled and said, *"If they've truly learned to listen to their body, that's my biggest success."*

That one line sums up who Anupama truly is – a coach who doesn't just transform bodies but helps you build a lifelong relationship with yourself.

S Abilash Nair

16. My Wellness Transformation: From the Road to Renewal

The Entrepreneur's Challenge

My name is R. Sathish Kumar, a 51-year-old entrepreneur based in Coimbatore, Tamil Nadu. My business involves educational equipment and digital transformation solutions, which requires extensive travel and constant customer visits. While I've always been conscious about my physical appearance, the demanding nature of my sales and marketing role often led to inconsistency in my fitness routine. For years, I operated under the flawed belief that eating heartily and exercising in parallel was the formula for good health. In reality, this approach resulted in a "bloated" physique that lacked true fitness, even though I wasn't technically overweight. My BMI was consistently on the border.

The COVID-19 lockdown in 2020 compounded the issue. With more time at home, our family indulged in self-cooked experiments, leading my weight to climb to 80 kgs. It was a clear sign that I needed a fundamental change.

A Life-Changing Conversation

During the uncertainty of the pandemic, I began calling relatives and friends more frequently. A conversation with my cousin, K. Anupama Nair, quickly deviated from the pandemic to the more pressing topics of mental wellness and health.

She introduced me to the concept of Intermittent Fasting (IF). The explanation was an eye-opener, and I decided to start practicing it immediately.

The Power of Intermittent Fasting

The initial days of fasting were tough, but I committed to the practice. Within six months, I had successfully dropped my weight from 80 kgs to 71 kgs. The physical change was rewarding, but the unexpected benefit was a profound feeling of mind, body, and soul alignment. Fasting taught me a discipline that extended beyond diet, helping to align my character and approach to life.

Encouraged by my success with the standard 16:8 IF schedule, I learned about more advanced protocols from Anupama, including the 20:4 Warrior Fasting and OMAD (One Meal a Day). I began practicing 20:4, which significantly boosted my confidence in my physical and mental endurance. On her advice, I also started hitting the gym, realizing that working out during the fasting window enhanced the positive effects.

Discipline for the Long Run

Today, I continue to practice these principles, primarily following the 16:8 fasting schedule and making it a point to avoid food after sunset.

For an entrepreneur like me, this physical and mental alignment has been invaluable. I can focus better on my profession, and my decision-making powers have noticeably increased, adding significant value to my business.

I am deeply thankful to my proud sister, K. Anupama Nair, for her guidance and for teaching me a sustainable practice that I believe will protect my health for the rest of my life. I am now hyper-aware of what I eat, and my body signals guide me with proper discipline.

I wish Anupama all the success in her mentoring journey, as I firmly believe that mental and physical wellness are the most important assets in today's world.

R Sathish Kumar

17. The Power of Showing Up: How I Reclaimed My Body and Mind

Thirteen years ago, before my son was born, fitness was woven seamlessly into the fabric of my daily life. Golf, yoga, half marathons, and a balanced diet weren't obligations—they were simply part of who I was. But as the demands of parenthood and career intensified, my well-established routine began to erode.

While I maintained my yoga practice, my relationship with food grew erratic. A troubling pattern emerged: I would commit to exercise for six or seven months each year, only to spend the remainder caught in a destructive cycle of overindulgence and rationalization. I told myself that doing well "most of the year" was enough.

The COVID-19 pandemic became an unexpected proving ground. During those uncertain months, I found focus again, aligning both my exercise regimen and dietary habits. Yet even then, the familiar barrier remained—I couldn't sustain my efforts beyond that six or seven-month threshold.

Everything shifted over the past three years when my partner helped me reframe my perspective entirely. I began viewing my body not as something to be occasionally maintained, but as a temple worthy of consistent investment and care.

In 2025, I made a decisive commitment to transform my relationship with health. Since May, I have:

- Exercised five to six days per week without exception
- Approached food with mindfulness and intentionality
- Learned to decline temptations while remaining fully present at social gatherings
- Developed the confidence to stand by my choices when others questioned my discipline

The transformation has been profound.

Eight months ago, the simple act of squatting and standing required considerable effort. Today, I cycle 60 kilometers, run 10 kilometers, and swim regularly—accomplishments I had never achieved in my entire life, all made possible through just four months of unwavering consistency.

This is no longer a temporary phase or another attempt. This is who I am now.

Finally, and more importantly, I remain deeply grateful to Anupama Nair, whose guidance I trust implicitly. Her approach is refreshingly straightforward —practical, sustainable methods that require only one thing from me—to show up.

What once felt like an insurmountable challenge has now become second nature. Consistency is no longer something I strive for; it is simply how I live.

Neha Bhatia

18. Sustainable Transformation: How Simple, Practical Guidance Led to Lasting Change

I was introduced to Anupama by my sister, who's a friend of hers, and I'm so glad I decided to connect. I had always tried to eat "healthy," but never really understood how to build a truly balanced meal. Anupama helped me break that down in such a simple, practical way – teaching me how to combine the right proportions of carbs, protein, and vegetables to fit my lifestyle and preferences.

What I appreciated most was how approachable her plans were. They weren't restrictive or complicated – just realistic, flexible, and easy to follow even with a busy schedule. In the early weeks, she was always available to answer my questions or suggest alternatives, which really helped me stay consistent.

Over time, I lost more than 20 lbs, but the real change has been in how I think about food. I've learned to listen to my body, make better choices, and maintain balance without feeling like I'm on a "diet." Even though I don't follow the plan strictly anymore, the habits she helped me build have truly transformed the way I eat and feel.

Anant Handa

In Closing...

You are not broken.

You are not behind.

You are not "too old," "too late," or "too busy."

You're just **one aligned decision away** from starting something powerful.

"Fat loss is not the goal. Feeling good, sleeping deep, moving freely – that's the real reward."

If you need a guide, I'm here.

But most importantly – you now have the tools to be your **own coach**.

Let's Begin Your Transformation

Take your measurements today

Commit to 3 months

Track the wins

Celebrate the shifts – inside and out

You've got this. And I've got your back.

Anupama Nair

Fat Loss & Gut Reset Coach

Founder, Sustainability Health Hub

From one seeker to another,

I see you. I believe in you.

And I promise — the version of you that you dream of?

That person is already within you.

About the Author

Anupama Nair is a certified fat loss and gut reset coach with a passion for helping high-achieving men & women reclaim their health, energy, and confidence – without crash diets or relentless gym routines.

Once a professional juggling career, motherhood, and family expectations, Anupama found herself trapped in a cycle of late nights, quick fixes, and burnout. Her turning point came not from a dramatic diagnosis, but from a deep realization: she had placed everything above her own well-being. What followed was not just a physical transformation, but a soulful journey from self-neglect to self-leadership.

Drawing from her personal health journey, Ayurvedic wisdom, and evidence-based nutrition, Anupama has coached over 2,000 men & women across the globe. She is known for blending science, simplicity, and empathy – helping them thrive with tools like intermittent fasting, habit stacking, somatic practices, and mindful eating.

A proud army daughter, devoted mother, and wife to a man who casually introduced her to intermittent fasting (and accidentally changed her life), Anupama now lives her purpose: to guide others from survival mode to sustainable wellness — one habit at a time.

This book is her story — and yours, if you're ready.